A Guide to Balancing Menopause: Thrive with menopause, and rediscover your younger self

Ron T. Baughman

Table of Contents:

INTRODUCTI ON

Embracing Menopause Excursion

Welcome to another part of your life! Menopause is a characteristic change that each lady encounters, denoting the finish of the regenerative years and the start of another stage. It's a period of progress, both truly and inwardly, and understanding the three phases of menopause can assist you to embrace

this excursion with certainty
and elegance. We should dig into an aide that will walk you through \
these stages and engage you to explore this extraordinary time effortlessly.

Stage 1: Perimenopause - A Preface to Change

Perimenopause fills in as the lead-up to menopause, similar to a
delicate preface to the orchestra of change. During this stage, which
can traverse numerous years, your chemical levels begin to change,
and you might see abnormalities in your monthly cycle. A few normal
side effects incorporate hot blazes, mind-set

swings, and changes in
rest designsDread not! Consider perimenopause as an amazing chance
to pay attention to your body and investigate better approaches to
sustain yourself. It's a chance to focus on taking care of oneself,
embrace better way of life propensities, and look for help from friends
and family or medical services experts who can direct you through this
change. Keep in mind, you're in good company on this excursion, and
numerous ladies track down solace in associating with other people

who are encountering comparable changes.

Stage 2: Menopause - Embracing Your New Ordinary

Menopause is formally acknowledged when a period has been missing for twelve successive months. While saying goodbye to your month to month cycles might summon blended feelings, menopause delivers additional opportunities and a feeling of freedom. It's a chance to commend the insight, certainty, and flexibility that accompany age.During menopause, you might experience side effects, for

example, hot flushes, night sweats, vaginal dryness, or changes in
mind-set. In any case, don't allow these side effects to eclipse the
positive parts of this stage. Embrace the newly discovered independence from contraception, find new interests, and set out on an
excursion of self-revelation. Keep in mind, menopause implies not a
closure, but rather the start of a new and energetic section in your life.

Stage 3: Post-menopause - Proceeding with your Excursion

Present menopause alludes to the years following
menopause,

described by security and self-disclosure. Your chemical levels have

settled, and you might notice a decrease in specific menopausal side effects. Nonetheless, It stays vital to focus on your general prosperity.

Center around keeping a sound way of life, including standard activity, adjusted nourishment, and taking care of oneself practices. Remain associated with your medical services supplier to screen bone

wellbeing, cardiovascular health, and generally imperativeness.

Post-menopause offers an amazing chance to embrace your

womanhood, seek after your interests, and set out on new undertakings.Menop ause is a characteristic and wonderful progress, notwithstanding its difficulties. By grasping the three phases - perimenopause, menopause, and post-menopause - you can explore this excursion with warmth, certainty, and self esteem. Keep in mind, each lady's experience is special, and embracing your singularity is fundamental as you leave on this new section. Thus, embrace the changes, look for help, and step in the right direction into this

Extraordinary excursion cheerfully and a spring in your step!

CHAPTER 1:

WHAT IS MENOPAUSE

Grasping the Rudiments

At the point when a lady for all time quits having feminine periods, she has arrived at the phase of life called menopause.

Frequently called the difference throughout everyday life, this stage flags the finish of a lady's capacity to have youngsters.

Numerous medical services suppliers really utilize the term

menopause to allude to the timeframe when a lady's chemical levels begin to change. Menopause is supposed to be finished when feminine periods have stopped for one ceaseless year.

The change stage before menopause is frequently alluded to as perimenopause. During this change time before menopause, the stock of mature eggs in a lady's ovaries reduces and ovulation becomes sporadic.

Simultaneously, the creation of estrogen and progesterone diminishes. It is the enormous drop in estrogen levels that causes the greater part of the side effects of menopause.

When does menopause happen?

Albeit the typical period of menopause is 51, menopause can really happen whenever from the 30s to the mid-50s or later. Ladies who smoke and are underweight will generally have a prior menopause, while ladies who are overweight frequently have a later menopause.

For the most part, a lady will in general have menopause at about as old as her mom did. Menopause can likewise occur because of reasons other than normal reasons. These include:

Untimely
menopause.
Untimely menopause
might happen when
there is ovarian
disappointment
before the age of 40.
It could be related
with smoking,
radiation openness,
chemotherapeutic
medications, or
medical procedures
that hinders the
ovarian blood
supply. Untimely
ovarian
disappointment is
likewise called
essential ovarian
deficiency.
Careful menopause.
Careful menopause
might follow the
evacuation of one or
the two ovaries, or
radiation of the
pelvis, including the
ovaries, in
premenopausal
ladies. This results in
an unexpected

menopause. These ladies frequently have more serious menopausal side effects than if they somehow managed to normally have menopause.Menopause is the point at which your period stops forever. Menopause is an ordinary piece of a lady's life. It is some of the time called "the difference throughout everyday life." Menopause doesn't occur at the same time. As your body advances to menopause more than quite a long while, you might have menopause side effects and unpredictable periods. The typical age for menopause in the US is 52. Perimenopause (PER-ee-MEN-gracious pawz), or the menopausal change, is the time paving the way to your last period. Perimenopause signifies "around menopause." Perimenopause is a long progress to menopause, or when your periods stop forever and you can never again get pregnant. As your body advances to menopause, your chemical levels might change haphazardly, causing menopause side effects suddenly. During this change, your ovaries make various measures of the chemicals estrogen (ES-teh-jin) and progesterone (proh-JES-tuh-RONE) than expected.Unpredictable periods occur during this time since you may not ovulate consistently. Your periods might be longer or more limited than expected. You could skirt a couple of months or have curiously lengthy or short feminine cycles. Your period might be heavier or lighter than previously.Numerous ladies additionally have hot blazes and other menopause side effects during this change. At the point when a lady has had no periods for 12 sequential months she is viewed as "postmenopausal". Most ladies become menopausal normally between the ages of 45 and 55 years, with the typical time of beginning at about 50 years. "Untimely menopause" may happen before the age of 40 because of either normal ovarian capability stopping, following a medical procedure to eliminate the ovaries, or because of disease therapies.

Menopause is thought of "ahead of schedule" when it happens somewhere in the range of 40 and 45 years.

CHAPTER 2

MENOPAUSE

SIDE EFFECTS

What is in store

1. Hot glimmers

Hot glimmers are among the most widely recognized side effects of menopause. They make somebody out of nowhere become hot, sweat-soaked, and flushed, particularly in the face, neck, and chest. A few females likewise experience chills.

2. Night sweats

Night sweats are hot glimmers that happen around evening time. Researchers don't know why they happen, but rather falling estrogen levels can influence the nerve center, which manages internal heart level

3. Sporadic periods

All through the menopausal change, having unpredictable or missed periods is typical. At last, a female will quit having periods completely.

4. Mind-set changes

Mind-set changes are capricious changes in temperament that are not connected with life-altering situations. They can make somebody feel abruptly miserable, teary, or furious. Mind-set changes are normal during perimenopause and menopause.

5. Bosom touchiness

Bosom delicacy is one more typical side effect of menopause, however its recurrence will in general diminish in the later stages.

6. Diminished drive

Menopause likewise usually influences charisma or longing for sex. This can be the immediate consequence of having lower levels of testosterone and estrogen, which can make actual excitement more troublesome.

Notwithstanding, it can likewise be an optional consequence of different side effects of menopause, for example, state of mind changes, or a symptom of a prescription.

7. Vaginal dryness

As female sex chemicals guarantee that there is a decent course of blood around the vagina, an absence of them can diminish the bloodstream and, in this manner, normal oil. This might cause dryness, which can be awkward or make penetrative sex more troublesome.

8. Cerebral pains
Somebody entering menopause might encounter more continuous cerebral pains or headache episodes because of a plunge in estrogen. This can be like the migraines that a few females experience before a period. However, dissimilar to during an ordinary monthly cycle, chemical levels during perimenopause can

vary all the more capriciously.

9. Shivering limits

During menopause, a few females experience shivering in the hands, feet, arms, and legs. This side effect is the consequence of chemical changes influencing the focal sensory system and regularly just goes on for a couple of moments all at once.

10. Consuming mouth

A consuming mouth is one more possible side effect of menopause and may show as a sensation of consuming, delicacy, shivering heat, or desensitization in or around the mouth.

This is one more aftereffect of hormonal changes. The bodily fluid chemicals in the mouth engage in sexual relations chemical receptors, which decline with a decrease in estrogen. This can add to agony and uneasiness.

11. Changes in taste

A few females might see changes in their feeling of taste, with more grounded flavors, during menopause. They may likewise encounter a dry mouth, which can prompt a higher gamble of creating gum sickness or holes.

12. Exhaustion

Exhaustion can be an upsetting and in some cases crippling menopause side effect. This could be the consequence of lower quality rest because of hot blazes and night sweats or the aftereffect of hormonal variances themselves.

13. Swelling

Females can encounter bulging during menopause for various reasons. They might encounter water maintenance, gassiness, or slow processing because of stress. If they change their dietary patterns close to this time, they may likewise encounter bulging.

14. Other stomach-related changes
Female sex chemicals impact the organisms an individual has in their mouth and gastrointestinal system. This can mean that during menopause, a female's stomach verdure changes in organization. They might see changes in their assimilation or they respond diversely to specific food sources.

15. Joint agony
Estrogen helps decline aggravation and keep the joints greased up. Subsequently, a few females experience joint torment because

of diminished estrogen.

Estrogen is answerable for managing liquid levels all through the body, so when the body turns out to be low in this chemical, females are more inclined to joint hurts or menopausal joint pain.

16. Muscle pressure and throbs

Females going through perimenopause or menopause can likewise encounter muscle pressure or throbs. This is because of similar variables as menopausal joint agony.

17. Electric shock sensations

Females can encounter impressions that look like electric shocks during perimenopause and menopause. It isn't clear what causes this, yet it very well might be the aftereffect of changing chemical levels in the sensory system.

18. Irritation

Since estrogen is connected with collagen creation and skin hydration, a decrease in this chemical can prompt expanded irritation or dryness, both around the vulva and somewhere else in the body.

19. Rest unsettling influence

A female's rest can become lighter or upset for some reasons during menopause. They might wake up often because of night sweats, get up prior, or find it hard to get to rest.

20.   Trouble concentrating

A decrease in estrogen can some of the time cause mental fogginess or trouble concentrating. Hot glimmers and rest issues may likewise be contributing variables.

21. Memory slips

Likewise, with fixation and concentration, menopause can influence memory.

Once more, this could be an immediate consequence of lower estrogen levels or compromised rest.

22. Diminishing hair

During menopause, hair misfortune or diminishing is one more aftereffect of ovarian hormonal vacillations. This makes the hair follicles contract, implying that hair develops all the more leisurely and sheds all the more without any problem.

23. Fragile nails

During or after menopause, the body may not deliver sufficient keratin, which is the substance that nails need major areas of strength to remain. This can prompt fragile, powerless nails that break or break without any problem.

24. Weight gain

Females can put on weight because of various components during menopause. A decrease in estrogen can bring about weight gain, as can bring down measures of actual work. Temperament changes can likewise imply that a female eats in an unexpected way

25. Stress incontinence

Stress incontinence alludes to an incessant or unexpected inclination to pee.

Certain individuals likewise allude to it as an overactive bladder.

This side effect is normal during menopause, as changes in chemical levels can make the bladder and pelvic muscles more vulnerable.

26. Mixed-up spells

The hormonal changes that happen during menopause influence insulin creation, which can make it challenging for the body to keep up with glucose solidness. This is the primary explanation that a few females experience mixed-up spells during perimenopause and menopause.

27. Sensitivities

Report new or deteriorating sensitivity side effects when they experience menopause. This happens because, during menopause, females can have spikes in receptors. The fact that it causes unfavorably susceptible responses makes the receptor synthetic.

28. Osteoporosis

During perimenopause, a decrease in estrogen can likewise bring about a deficiency of bone thickness. In serious cases, this can prompt osteoporosis, which makes the bones more delicate and break without any problem.

29. Unpredictable heartbeat

A few females might encounter an unpredictable heartbeat, or arrhythmia, during or after menopause. It is in every case best to examine side effects connecting with the heart with a specialist.

30. Stench

Hot glimmers and night sweats can bring about an expansion in personal stench during menopause. Assuming a female frequently feels worried or restless, they may likewise see that they are perspiring more.

31. Crabbiness

Either because of hormonal vacillations or the effect of other menopause side effects, females going through this change might find that they feel crabby. Stress or an absence of rest may likewise add to this.

32. Discouragement

For certain females, hormonal irregular characteristics might set off gloom. Nonetheless, for this situation, sadness is frequently situational and may not be a long haul. An absence of rest and stress can add to this. At times, menopause might set off discouragement or a low state of mind in light of the change it implies in a female's life. Any critical life-altering event can assume a part in wretchedness, regardless of whether the change is a positive one.

33. Uneasiness

Uneasiness is another state of mind-related side effect that a few females experience during menopause. It might deteriorate around

evening time or just happen discontinuously as chemical levels vacillate.

Likewise, with menopause-related sadness, this nervousness might be situational and improve once chemicals level out

34. Alarm jumble

Now and again, females might encounter fits of anxiety during menopause. At the point when these assaults happen startlingly or out of nowhere, they can show alarm jumble. This might occur because of hormonal changes or the anxiety toward feeling restless.

CHAPTER 3

MANAGING

MOOD AND

MIND

Handling Emotional Change

1. Keep A Journal

Keeping a side effect journal, recording your side effects every day, will help wellbeing experts to evaluate whether your low state of mind has a repetitive, hormonal premise or whether you might be experiencing melancholy which ought to be dealt with in an unexpected way. A few ladies in their

40s are endorsed antidepressants for low temperament however these can have undesirable secondary effects while chemical substitution treatment (HRT) is a more compelling and more secure treatment for mind-set swings set off bychanges.

2. Take Some HRT

In the UK, HRT (which includes taking estrogen with a progestogen for ladies who actually have their bellies) is prescribed by Good to treat menopause-related state of mind swings and examination has shown it makes a difference. One review, distributed prior this year[2018] by US scientists, found ladies who took HRT for a year were less inclined to foster side effects of sadness during the menopause.There are a few dangers related with taking HRT yet these are tiny and the advantages offset the dangers. The sort and portion of HRT will rely upon your singulair side effects and clinical history with the counsel of your PCP.

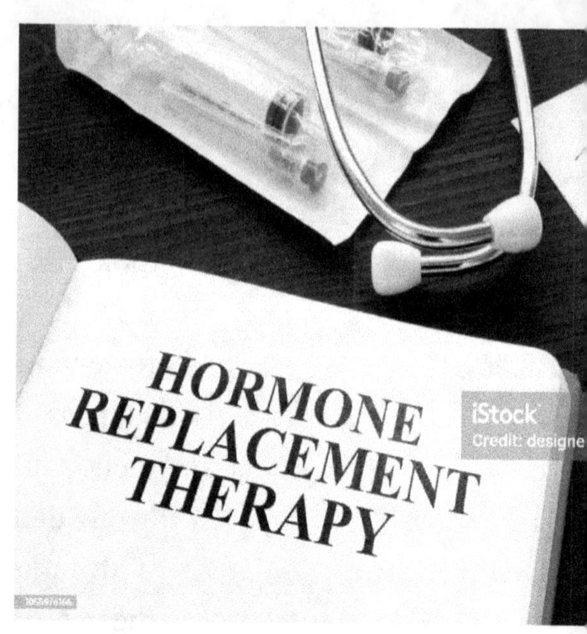

3   .Attempt testosterone

A few ladies with low moxie are recommended a testosterone gel to use close by HRT. Low state of mind can be exacerbated by low moxie, sexual brokenness and issues in your relationship and utilizing modest quantities of testosterone gel might support your charisma and energy levels, thus assisting with further developing temperament. Your singular case should be surveyed by a specialist and a low portion is normally recommended at first

4. Eat Well

Eating strongly may work on your temperament while devouring a lot of caffeine or sweet food varieties could prompt pointless ups and downs of energy levels. Some proof that lack specific nutrients, like B12 and magnesium, can influence your state of mind so expanding your admission of eating slick fish, rich in omega-3, may likewise further develop the mindset.Food sources high in estrogen-like mixtures called phytoestrogens, for example, soybeans, lentils, and heartbeats may likewise be beneficial. Some examination has shown that Japanese ladies, who have an eating routine high in phytoestrogens, experience fewer menopausal side effects than ladies on a Western eating routine.

5. Scale-Back Liquor

Although at first liquor goes about as an energizer, it in the end has a calming, burdensome impact, so standard, heavy drinking can cause you to feel down. Drinking with some restraint and declining for a few days or seven days ought to affect your temperament.

6.   Work-out Routinely

A few examinations show that individuals who work out routinely are more joyful. It isn't clear precisely why - it may be the case that better individuals essentially feel improved or that exercise might emphatically affect cerebrum science. Exercise can likewise work on your rest and confidence when menopausal ladies might have a humiliated outlook on their side effects or stress over maturing.Exercises, for example, a dance class, taking up tennis or joining an activity class are friendly as well as, as they include weight-bearing activity, will assist with combatting the adverse consequences of the menopause on bone well being.

7. Get More Rest

Everybody realizes that feeling tired makes us tired. Embracing procedures to work on the sum and nature of your rest could support your mindset.

8. Think about Corresponding Treatments

Chemical substitution treatment (HRT) has been all the more completely explored and demonstrated to be more viable than the other options, although reciprocal treatments can in any case be a valuable choice based on your singulair side effects.Some exploration recommends that the homegrown cure of St John's Wort can assist with easing emotional episodes, even though it can connect with other medicines, so it merits examining every one of the choices with a medical care professional first.

9. Take a stab at A genuinely new thing. Going through menopause can coincide with an unpleasant time in ladies' lives with changing conditions, for example, kids venturing out from home or stress over progressing in years. These could be an ideal opportunity to find another job that will fulfill you, for example, getting back to work, chipping in, enlisting on a course, which will work on your

confidence   and
mindset.

CHAPTER 4

REMAINING

SOUND

Exercise,Diet,Rest

Exercise

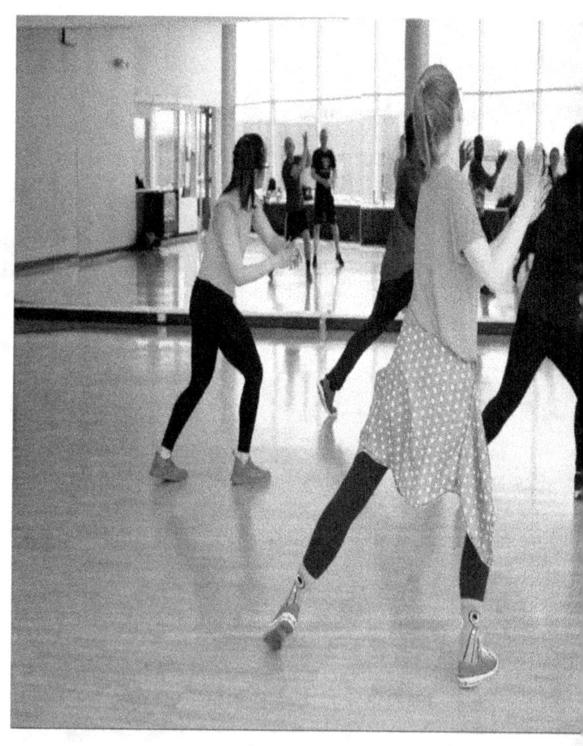

Practices that can
help ,Two primary

kinds of activity are suggested for menopausal ladies - vigorous activity and strength preparation. High-impact practice is a cardio practice that expands your pulse and utilizes enormous muscle gatherings.Sorts of high-impact practice include,

Strolling - This is the easiest type of low-effect vigorous activity and consumes calories when performed at an energetic speed.

Swimming - Another low-influence cardio exercise that is simpler on the joints than different exercises like running.

Moving An extraordinarily vigorous exercise that is low-influence, consumes calories, and when joined with mixing Latin rhythms as in Zumba can be loads of fun too!.Whether it's strolling, swimming, moving, running, or bicycle riding, you ought to begin with light oxygen-consuming movement, especially if you have not practiced consistently for some time. Begin with 10 minutes per day, and slowly increase the force and duration of your activity as you feel yourself becoming fitter.Strength preparation is likewise suggested for ladies during and after menopause, as it's an incredible method for consuming calories, reinforcing muscles,and diminishing muscle-to-fat ratio. Kinds of solidarity preparing to incorporate weight machines, obstruction preparing, and hand-held loads. This kind of activity is especially significant for developing bone fortitude to assist with warding off osteoporosis, which turns into a more serious gamble when estrogen levels drop during menopause. While strength preparing, you ought to pick a weight or opposition level that tires out your muscles after around twelve reiterations, and afterward, progressively increment that level over the long haul as you feel yourself getting more grounded. You ought to expect to do three strength preparation exercises in seven days.

Practicing tips

Remember these tips on the off chance that you choose to begin an activity system during or after menopause:Attempt to do no less than 75

minutes of
overwhelming
oxygen-consuming
movement seven
days, or two times
that sum if by some
stroke of good luck
doing direct vigorous
activity.Ensure you
put forth sensible and
reachable objectives
for yourself, and
often change and
update your
everyday practice to
keep it from getting
lifeless,Attempt and
make your activity
system fun. You can

practice any place you are, and exercises like planting and yard work can likewise consider working out, and ensure you start with light activity from the beginning, and move toward additional lively exercises as you progress. Make certain to heat up and chill off when each activity.Active work is valuable in each phase of our lives. It works on our wellness, advances weight reduction, and keeps our hearts solid. Getting physical during and after menopause additionally has the additional advantage of assisting with counterbalancing sickness, and is likewise viewed as supportive in decreasing menopausal side effects like pressure, tension, and discouragement.

Diet

Nourishment assumes a fundamental part in your general well-being. All through perimenopause, menopause, and post-menopause, what you eat can likewise influence how you feel. Consolidating sugars, proteins, and food varieties high in calcium, vitamin K and vitamin D might assist with facilitating side effects during this change.

Carbs

Carbs are significant for energy and cerebrum capability. Weakness and memory issues are normal side effects during menopause, so it's fundamental for ladies to consume carbs that invigorate the body and cerebrum.Starches are one of the three essential supplements in food and one of your body's primary energy sources. There are three sorts of carbs:Sugars are the most essential type of carb. Sugars are normally fostered in many natural products, vegetables, and milk. Staying away from Food varieties with added sugars are ideal.Starches are mind-boggling carbs that the body separates into sugar to use for energy. Starch is in bread, pasta, potatoes, peas and corn.Fiber is another complex carb. High-fiber diets might assist with forestalling stomach and digestive issues. Food varieties high in fiber incorporate nuts, seeds, entire grains, and beans.

Proteins

Made of amino acids, protein is a supplement used to develop and fix cells.Famous protein sources incorporate meat, eggs, dairy items, seeds, and nuts."Protein is fundamentally important, yet not to the avoidance of any remaining things," says Dr. Huber. "There's a compelling reason to have a protein shake three times each day, yet attempt to ensure that you're getting protein consistently at most dinners and bites. It will assist with keeping glucose stable and is related to better bone thickness and diminished crack gamble.

Food sources High in Calcium

Individuals going through menopause ought to integrate calcium into their eating routine since it is fundamental for heart and bone well-being. During menopause, ladies ought to expect to get 1,200 milligrams of calcium, which is somewhat more than the 1,000 milligrams of calcium suggested for somebody not going through menopause. Individuals going through menopause ought to talk with their primary care physician about whether they're getting adequate calcium because of the hazard of osteoporosis. Dairy, similar to milk and cheddar, is one of the most well-known wellsprings of calcium. You can likewise get calcium from verdant greens like wavy kale and okra.

Food varieties High in Vitamin K and Vitamin D

Vitamin K and vitamin D work

together to work on
bone well-being,
fundamental for
those going through
menopause, as bone
thickness
diminishes during
this progress, makes
sense to Doyle.
Vitamin D and
vitamin K are
significant for
calcium retention
and to coordinate
calcium from
delicate tissues and
supply routes to
bones, separately.
Ladies in menopause
and postmenopause
ought to go for the
gold of
vitamin K, which is
about four to five
cups of salad greens,
and 800 to
900 IU of vitamin D
day to day, which
would be like a
salmon filet.
You can get vitamin
D from slick fish,

similar to salmon and sardines,
red meat, liver, and egg yolks. Incredible wellsprings of vitamin K incorporate dull salad greens, for example, kale, spinach, collard greens, and Brussels sprouts. The vast majority need vitamin D supplementation to keep up with sufficient levels. Converse with your primary care physician about what enhancements would be ideal to attempt.

Rest

Menopause might be inescapable, however, there are things ladies can do to further develop the best quality:
Work-out routinely

.

Stop smoking if you
smoke right now.
Nicotine can
adversely affect
rest.
Wear lightweight,
breathable cotton
garments when you
rest.
Wash up before bed.
Lay down with light
covers, not weighty
covers.
Utilize a fan or
cooling to further
develop airflow in
your room.
Stay away from
nicotine, liquor, or
potentially caffeine
before bed.
Practice pressure the
executive's
strategies, like
contemplation, back
rub, or yoga.
Eat quality feasts and
try not to eat a huge,
weighty supper. Be
aware
of any food varieties
that trigger hot

glimmers, like hot or acidic food sources.

Clinical mediation to further develop rest

If the way-of-life adjustments don't help, converse with your PCP about enhancements or chemical substitution therapy. Hormone substitution treatment. "Hormonally, progesterone straightforwardly affects rest and a few patients find that daily progesterone supplementation can further develop rest designs.

Melatonin has been displayed to help. Get your primary care

physician's OK
before taking any
new enhancements.
Converse with your
doctor assuming that
you experience
difficulty
resting, whether it's
connected with
menopause etc.
Persistent sleep
deprivation can
prompt hypertension,
coronary illness, and
other
serious ailments.

CHAPTER 5

EATING RIGHT

Sustenance Tips
There are seven
nutrients significant
during menopause
1. Eat leafy foods
first
Products of the soil
are among the best
food sources we can
eat. These

stalwart food sources
are loaded with
nutrients, minerals,
and products
of the soil and ought
to take up a portion
of your plate at
eating times.
Research has
connected many
advantages of eating
more products of
the soil intended for
menopausal ladies,
including:
Decreased hot
glimmer.
Better rest
Lower paces of
wretchedness
Further weight
reduction
Lower pulse
A study in 2000 even
found that broccoli
helped decline levels
of
estrogen related to
bosom malignant
growth and expanded
estrogen

levels that help
safeguard against
bosom disease.
Tip: Bite on entire
products of the soil
over the day or eat
leafy foods
first at eating times.
2. Add dairy to your
eating regimen
during menopause.
Milk ,yogurt, and
cheddar offer the
significant nutrients
and minerals
ladies need to battle
bone misfortune.
These fundamental
supplements
incorporate calcium,
phosphorus,
potassium,
magnesium, and
nutrients
D and K.
Tip: Tidbit on low-
fat yogurt with
granola or a natural
product, or
appreciate cheddar
and nuts as a
delectable evening
treat.

3. Work on your wellbeing with whole grains

Entire grains have been connected to numerous medical advantages, including a decreased chance of malignant growth, coronary illness, and, surprisingly, unexpected passing. Tip: Lift your entire grain consumption with basic trades. Utilize entire-grain pasta in a most loved recipe and switch sandwich bread from white to entire-grain. Make cereal in a sluggish cooker. Attempt earthy-colored rice or quinoa as a side.

4. All fats are not made equal.

Solid fats play a significant part in everybody's eating routine, particularly for ladies during menopause. These food varieties, including greasy fish, flax seeds, chia seeds, and avocados, can assist your body with the engrossing supplements it needs and may decrease the recurrence and seriousness of menopause side effects.

Tip: Get your fill of solid fats by sprinkling chia seeds in a smoothie, finishing off a sandwich with avocado, or eating fish two times every week

5. Eat quality protein

Protein can assist with supporting bulk and bone strength—two things that decay during menopause. Ongoing examination proposes that

more seasoned adults
may require more
than the suggested
sum for
adults north of 18.
This can assist with
decreasing the risk of
sarcopenia (the
deficiency of bulk,
strength, and
capability).
The best wellsprings
of sound protein
include:
Beans and vegetables
Wild salmon
Eggs
Greek yogurt
Converse with your
primary care
physician about how
much protein is
ideal for you. Excess
can influence your
well-being.
6. Limit handled
food sources
Handled food
sources are
commonly loaded
with salt and refined
sugar, the two of
which can adversely

influence your well-being.
High-salt food varieties can bring down a lady's bone thickness, and refined sugar can add superfluously to your waistline.
Tip: Make feasts and snacks early on to make helpful and quality food
That is not difficult to get in a hurry.
7. Get dynamic
Active work is great for each age and phase of life, and menopause is the same. Standard activity has been connected to numerous medical advantages for menopausal ladies, including:
More grounded bones
More grounded heart
More grounded muscles

Further developed
perseverance
A further developed
mindset
A better night's rest
Solid weight
Diminished hazards
of disease
Social associations
that help mental and
actual wellbeing
Tip: Request that a
companion go along
with you as you
make
progress toward 15
minutes of
moderately active
work consistently.

CHAPTER 6

REGULAR CURES

All-encompassing Methodologies
Plant food sources
With naturopathic
approaches, one
doesn't require

manufactured
synthetic treatment.
Essentially eating
more plant food
sources like
vegetables,
vegetables, natural
products, entire
grains,
nuts, and seeds can
offer some help, as
they contain
chemical adjusting
plant synthetic
compounds known
as phytoestrogens.
Ground flaxseeds
likewise contain
phytoestrogens and
have been displayed
in
examinations to
diminish hot
glimmers. In one
review, ladies had
hot
blaze help when they
consumed 40 grams
of ground flaxseeds
every
day. Aged soy food
varieties like tofu,

miso, and tempeh
can likewise
assist with lessening
hot blazes.
Spices
Spices can likewise
mitigate menopausal
side effects. Dark
cohosh has
been displayed in
various examinations
to free a large
number from
menopausal side
effects including hot
blazes, nervousness,
sleep
deprivation, heart
palpitations, and
sadness. Take 40-80
mg of a
normalized removal
every day.
Maca root has a rich
history of purpose in
Peru to help ladies
through
the menopausal
process. A few
twofold visually
impaired, fake
treatment-controlled
investigations

demonstrate the way
that it can be
sure to assist hot
glimmers and
various other
menopausal side
effects.
Take 1,000-2,000 mg
day to day.
Another exceptional
natural concentrate is
red clover. As
indicated by
research, this viable
elective treatment for
menopause attempts
to ease
hot glimmers,
vaginal dryness, and
uneasiness. Take 40
mg of a
concentrate two
times every day.
Vitex, otherwise
called a chaste berry,
helps normal
menopausal side
effects, for example,
hot glimmers and
night sweats, and is
likewise
powerful for
premenopausal side

effects like
unpredictable and
weighty periods. I
for the most part
suggest a normalized
concentration
80-240 mg every
day.
Also, think about
Pueraria Mirifica.
This individual from
the vegetable
 Family contains
chemical-adjusting
phytoestrogens. One
investigation
discovered that 50-
100 mg every day for
six days decreased
hot blazes
and night sweats.
Homeopathy
Try not to underrate
the viability of
homeopathic
solutions for the
decrease of
menopausal side
effects. One of the
most well-known
cures
is sweet Sepia. Side
effects that

recommend this cure
incorporate hot
glimmers, night
vaginal dryness,
touchiness, low
charisma, and
depletion. One more
,A typical solution
for consideration is
Pulsatilla.
Ladies who might
profit from this
homeopathic
medication feel
awful
in warm climates and
want natural air.
They might have
mindset
swings and
tearfulness and feel
improved
with organization.
They ordinarily
hunger for desserts
like chocolate.
**Regular
Antidepressants**
Assuming that you
are experiencing
uneasiness or gloom
with
menopause.

There is regular
assistance accessible.
Other than the
normal chemical
balancers previously
referenced, 5-
hydroxytryptophan,
known as
5-HTP,
may likewise be
valuable. It supports
the synapse serotonin
to loosen
up the mind and
advance a superior
state of mind. When
taken before
sleep time, it can
likewise assist with
lightening sleep
deprivation.
A common portion is
100 mg taken a few
times every day
while
starving.
**Test Your
Chemicals**
Chemical irregular
characteristics can
bring about hot
glimmers,

vaginaldryness and diminishing, night sweats, sleep deprivation, tipsiness, heart palpitations, migraines, memory issues, decreased drive, bladder and pee issues, mindset swings, misery, tension, exhaustion, and, surprisingly, joint agony. In a perfect world, it is ideal to go through a chemical test to figure out which chemical lopsided characteristics you might have, as they contrast with every lady and at various phases of menopause. For ladies with gentle-to-direct side effects of menopause, diet, workout, and healthful enhancements, particularly natural and homeopathic cures, are typically enough. The utilization of regular progesterone cream has all the earmarks of being extremely protected and compelling when a more grounded approach is required. Similarly, forerunner chemicals, for example,pregnenolone and DHEA, might be useful. For ladies with outrageous side effects that are lethargic to nourishing enhancements, the utilization of bio-indistinguishable chemical therapy* is exceptionally successful. This is especially valid for ladies who had their ovaries taken out at an

early age or others
with moderate-to-
serious osteoporosis.

CHAPTER 7

YOUR
SEXUALITY

Exploring Closeness

How would you keep
up with closeness
during menopause?
Ponder Sex. A lady's
cerebrum is as yet
her most significant
sexual organ.
Make a Private
Arrangement.
Compose sex on the
schedule. ...
Take an alternate
route from
Intercourse.
Imagination can be
sexual for
couples. ...
Search for Sex. …

Center around That
Body — Inside and
Out. ...
Make some noise. ...
Try not to Stop.
Recollecting the first
close-to-home
closeness
What was it about
your accomplice that
pulled you to them at
first? Do
you recollect? An
outing through a
world of fond
memories can assist
with recovering
sentiments that were
alive previously. It
can ship you
to a nostalgic overall
setting, help you to
remember what you
had, and
assist with
explaining what is as
yet conceivable.
Evoke times that
assist you with
feeling associated
with your
accomplice,
reinforce your

ongoing sentiments,
and resuscitate your
interest in them.
Recollect times you
snickered together or
perhaps pay attention
to the
music you used to
both appreciate - this
is one of the
speediest ways of
animating your
close-to-home
closeness and
bringing back good
sentiments!
**Rediscovering
shared needs**
Our central feelings
drive us as people
and fruitful
connections
relyupon shared
needs fulfillment. A
lot of what prompts
feeling
disengaged as far as
close-to-home
closeness is the point
at which we
don't see how to
satisfy our own or

each other's
requirements solidly
and practically.
Requirements could
incorporate well-
being and security,
offering and
getting
consideration,
feeling esteemed and
significant, and
feeling
known and
comprehended.
These requirements
are not debatable yet
the limits and cutoff
points on how you
meet them with one
another
Couples can pull out
from one another
when their
requirements go
neglected and end up
in a deadlock, both
reluctant to step
forward and
reestablish what has
eroded. It is entirely
expected to accept
you are

addressing your
accomplice's
requirements and
that they ought to
understand what you
want - yet
presumptions don't
push you ahead in
the manner that
genuine request and
interest do.
Thus, now is the
right time to
investigate what you
want to feel
associated with,
cherished, and
protected by posing a
few inquiries:
What is it that you
want?
What is it that your
accomplice needs?
Is your accomplice a
first concern?
Do every one of you
feel regarded and
esteemed?
What might be
occurring for you
both to feel these
necessities were
being met?

Tracking down
things to appreciate
The profound
closeness in a
relationship relies
upon the
concentration
and consideration
you give it. It's not
difficult to review
your
accomplice from a
perspective of
examination and
bothering when
untied in the riptide
of continuous
pressure and when
you may be
deficient with
regards to saving
close to home limit.
To assemble
association, you want
to make snapshots of
appreciation
and post for your
accomplice's
endeavors to
interface as well.
Notice
your accomplice
accomplishing

something positive,
but little, and offer
veritable
commendations and
certification. This
will assist with
setting
aside an installment
in the relationship's
financial balance and
empower a culture of
harmony.
Keep in mind, what
we could do without
is consistently
accessible yet
so is what we can
appreciate.
**Start valiant
correspondence**
It can take fortitude
to open up assuming
that the association
and
profound closeness
between two
individuals appears
to be stale or you
are feeling
defenseless. Truly
weakness is the
brilliant string that
winds

around a snare of
association with each
other when you can
perceive
each other's
uneasiness and
delicacy.
It requires facing
challenges however
can be loaded up
with wealth
androuse others to do
likewise. It can make
a more profound
comprehension of
each other and see
past the defensive
layer we can
protect ourselves
with.
Profound awareness
and previous
encounters can
expand our anxiety
toward being
harmed, deserted, or
misconstrued. The
mind is an
example of a
matching organ and
we can act in
receptive and
pointless

ways assuming that
there is a clue or sign
that makes us aware
of a
previous encounter
that has a difficult
close-to-home tag.
Having a
familiarity with what
your triggers are can
assist with bringing
them
into your
mindfulness and
empower you to
answer all the more
deliberately.
Begin with a little
and sensible
discussion that will
start to make the
propensity for being
more powerless and
limit the gamble of
becoming
enacted. This could
be as straightforward
as being willing to
show
good feelings around
your accomplice,
communicating
actual warmth,

or sharing how
profoundly you feel
about something.
As opposed to
considering this to be
possibly a triumph
on the off
chance that your
accomplice answers
in a way that meets
your
expectations and
assumptions, view it
as an approach to
reinforcing
portions of yourself
that will prompt
more development. It
is the
beginning of
building an extension
to one another's
hearts and reviving
profound closeness.
The most effective
method to increment
actual closeness in a
relationship.
Any everyday issue
that you need to
foster necessitates
some

purposeful activity.
If your relationship is
at the lower part of
the plan
for the day and
without food, it will
rot after some time.
Closeness can
become dulled with
the lowly, dreariness
of a homegrown
daily
practice, so you
should know about
how you are
enhancing your
relationship. Starting
to set out customs
gives freedom to do
this.
Ceremonies are
rehashed approaches
to drawing in with
one another
that convey a
positive profound
part that recognizes
them from
everyday practice.
They can be little yet
the aggregate impact
is
powerful.

Take a stab at setting
up a few delicate
ceremonies that are
not difficult
to do and develop the
propensity for
chuckling, liveliness,
and contact:.
Investigate by
leaving some
adoration notes or
sending some
coquettish messages.
Focus on being
available to one
another by halting to
welcome each
other appropriately
consistently or after
supper.
Consider a couple of
moments of
interfacing
discussion instead of
critical thinking
about any issues
The sizzle of
physical allure will
be a recurring pattern
however
fellowship, regard,
fun, and cherishing

expectation,
alongside the
thoughts above, can
navigate the way to
activity to decidedly
reestablish closeness
and erotic nature. Be
inventive and put
your
creative mind and
recover that
cherishing, exotic
inclination.

CHAPTER 8

**ADJUSTING LIFE
Stress, Taking care
of oneself, and
Objectives
Stress**
Our body produces
two chemicals under
pressure: adrenaline
and
cortisol.
They are otherwise
called your 'flight or
flight' chemicals.
Delivered in
the adrenal organs,
adrenaline builds

your pulse and
circulatory strain
and lifts energy,
while cortisol
increments glucose
levels. Cortisol
likewise modifies
insusceptible
framework reactions
and smothers the
stomach-related and
conceptual
frameworks.
When the pressure
passes, your
chemical levels drop,
and your body
gets back to its not-
unexpected state. Be
that as it may, long-
haul
(constant Stress can
upset practically all
of your body's
cycles.
Uneasiness, high
sugar, and struggle at
home or work can
prompt the
adrenal organs to
support elevated
degrees of cortisol,
which can

prompt gloom,
weariness, cerebral
pains, a sleeping
disorder, and
mental haze.
Persistent pressure
can likewise expand
the risk of
strokes, diabetes, and
cardiovascular
failures.
Expanded cortisol
levels additionally
influence the
development of
estrogen and
progesterone. During
perimenopause, the
adrenal organs
assume control over
the development of
estrogen. Assuming
the
adrenal organs are
making pressure
chemicals, they
probably won't
have the option to
make estrogen and
progesterone.

**Effect of weight on
menopause side
effects**

Hot flushes can be
set off by pressure as
it comes down on
our sensory
system.
Rest issues emerge
as low estrogen
influences our
capacity to get to
rest and/or stay
unconscious long
enough to get a
decent night's rest.
Stress can rapidly
worsen on the off
chance that you lie in
bed stressing
around evening .
Mind-set swings can
be set off by pressure
as we stress over
things
more or feel
incapable of adapting
Weight gain can
increase as your
body tracks down
alternate ways of
expanding estrogen
creation by putting
away fat around the
stomach.

We likewise will
quite often need
sweet or undesirable
food varieties
when we are focused
on that can increase
exhaustion as well as
weight
gain.
Stomach-related
inconveniences
emerge when you are
focused on that
can prompt
heartburn, bulging,
obstruction and leave
you feeling
commonly awkward
**Taking care of
oneself**
Way of life and
sustenance changes
can assist with
dealing with your
sensations of stress.
Take on these
beneficial routines to
assist you with
combating pressure:
Thump the persistent
vices. It is vital to
stay away from
undesirable

approaches to
overseeing pressure,
for example, utilizing
liquor,
smoking, or solace
eating.
Keep away from
handled food sources
and high-sugar-
counting
calories.
Your body utilizes
cortisol to bring your
glucose levels back
up after
cake and espresso, so
expect to keep your
glucose levels
adjusted.
Balance your eating
regimen. Partaking in
an improved eating
regimen
with different
vegetables will fight
off the desires of
unfortunate food
sources.
Great-quality protein
with lean meat, slick
fish, eggs, and
heartbeats

will assist in keeping
you full longer.
Remain hydrated.
Make sure to hydrate
with non-charged
liquids over
the day; go for 2
liters per day.
Move more. Partake
in any exercises that
get your pulse up and
fortify
your muscles; this
could be moving,
lively strolling,
running, yoga, or
weightlifting.
What's more,
unwind. Set aside a
few minutes for side
interests like
perusing, paying
attention to music,
expressions, and
specialties, or
cultivating. Consider
or keep a diary to
record your
considerations or
what you're thankful
for.
**Taking care of
oneself: tips**

1. Keep a period
schedule
During
perimenopause,
feminine cycles start
to change. Cycles
can get
longer or more
limited, and streams
can be heavier or
lighter. Keeping
a schedule of your
cycles can assist you
with following
changes and
sorting out your new
typical (for an
extraordinary method
for doing
this, look at the
cycle-following in
the schedule segment
of the Ovia
Richness
application!).
A schedule is
likewise useful if you
have different kinds
of feedback
you need to impart to
your primary care
physician.

2. Deal with your
bones
The risk of bone
misfortune
(osteoporosis) goes
up around
menopause.
So this moment is an
incredible
opportunity to begin
dealing with your
bone wellbeing. This
is how you might
keep your bones
solid:
Add wellsprings of
calcium and vitamin
D to your eating
routine.
Try not to smoke,
and drink with some
restraint.
Get a standard
weight-bearing,
strength-preparing,
and balance
workout.
Weight-bearing and
strength practices put
weight on your
bones, which
increments bone
mass. Go for the gold

of activity
somewhere multiple
times every week.
Balance practices
safeguard your bones
by
decreasing your risk
of falling.
3. Adhere to a sound
weight
Numerous ladies
begin putting on
weight in the years,
making a
beeline for and after
menopause,
particularly around
the midsection.
Since stomach fat
might raise your risk
of coronary illness,
it's smart to
watch out for weight
gain. Think about
making a move to
zero in on
eating great and
setting aside a few
minutes for a
workout. What's
more, talk with your
PCP about the

weight that is smart
for you.
4. Safeguard your
rest
A few ladies make
some harder
memories getting a
decent night's rest
around menopause,
so consider stepping
up your rest
propensities.
Have a go at saving a
period before bed
every night to
accomplish
something quiet and
loosening up that sets
you in the right state
of
mind to relinquish
the day.
You can likewise
work on your rest by
keeping a standard
rest plan,
ensuring your room
is cool and dim, and
skipping liquor,
caffeine, and
weighty dinners for a
couple of hours
before sleep time.

If hot glimmers
(otherwise called
night sweats) are
intruding on your
rest,
There are loads of
things that can help.
Learn about
medicines here.
5. Give your teeth
and gums some
adoration
Did you have at least
some idea that gum
sickness builds your
gamble
for coronary illness?
It's only another
motivation to take
great
consideration of your
mouth, including
day-to-day brushing
and
flossing, alongside
dental specialist
visits two times
every year.
6. Sustain your skin
Sound skin isn't just
about cleaning
agents and creams.
To keep your

skin shining, abstain
from smoking, lower
pressure, get
sufficient rest
and actual work, and
drink a lot of water
— that's right,
basically every
one of the significant
things that assist with
keeping the
remainder of
your body well, as
well. It's likewise
essential to routinely
utilize
sunscreen. Assuming
your skin is dry, skirt
hot showers and
showers
since they can dry
your skin much
more.
7. Remember your
Kegels
You could recall
Kegels assuming
you've at any point
been pregnant,
and they're
significant again
now. That is because
urinary incontinence

is normal around
menopause and then
some. Kegels can
help by
reinforcing your
pelvic floor — and
you can do them
essentially
whenever and
anyplace. Contract
the muscles you use
when you pee,
hold, and deliver.
Pursue 10 Kegels,
five times each day.
(One extraordinary
result of
Kegels: they can
further develop your
sexual coexistence,
as well.)
8. Take care of your
heart
There are parts you
can do to keep your
heart solid and lower
your
gamble for
cardiovascular
illness. Furthermore,
assuming you're as of
now intending to
attempt the taking

care of oneself
propensities above,
you take care of the
greater part of the
solid heart list:
9.Get normal
activity.
1o..Keep your
weight in the sound
reach.
11.Eat well,
including a lot of
natural products,
veggies, protein, and
entire grains
12.Lower pressure.
13.Abstain from
smoking. (We realize
that stopping is one
of the
hardest ways of life
transforms you can
make. Converse with
your PCP
about ways of
making a difference.)
14.Have your
circulatory strain
checked, and work
with your PCP
assuming that your
numbers are high.

15.Have your
cholesterol and fatty
substances checked,
and make
changes to your
eating regimen or
start a prescription
assuming that
your numbers are
over the solid reach.
Objectives
Fortunately, as
objective-situated
ladies, we can utilize
the abilities
We've fabricated and
sharpened our games
to handle this new
test.
1. Observe Yourself!

It requires a ton of
investment, energy,
and devotion to work
out
routinely or
potentially get
yourself to the
beginning lines.
Indeed,
even among the
individuals who can,

relatively few work
out
consistently. On the
off chance that you
consistently do
perseverance
and strength
workouts, you're in a
significantly more
modest minority.
Around 15% of
ladies in nations
routinely participate
in the base
measures of
solidarity and
cardiovascular
activity. Your most
A memorable
objective is to step
back and give
yourself props.
2. Track down a
clinical partner.
Your PCP ought to
be a partner in your
dynamic life. If that
is not the
best situation for
you, this moment's
the opportunity to
find a specialist

who comprehends
athletic people.'You
need to quit doing
that. It's only
excessively risky for
somebody your age.'
I said, 'All things
considered, you don't
have any idea who
you're conversing
with.
Furthermore, this is
the last time we'll be
speaking.' The
clinical calling
doesn't manage
competitors a ton.
Somebody with a
clinical game
foundation will say,
'Good, do this and
this, and continue
onward."
3. Join a steady
gathering
Cerebrum haze, hot
glimmers, gloom…
we as a whole are
going
through menopause
difficulties and no
one comprehends
that very like

other dynamic ladies going through them. Alongside working with your PCP, track down a gathering of similar ladies to share battles and possible arrangements. It assists you with knowing you're in good company and can move you to handle new difficulties.

4..Apply your development mentality.
As competitors and dynamic ladies, we're continuously pursuing objectives and inquiring, "What's straightaway"? At the point when we hit the obstacles of menopause or the progressions that can accompany

absolute aging, we
can begin looking in
reverse as opposed to
advance. That won't
be exceptionally
useful or supportive.
Rather than
attempting to
contrast now with
then, at that point, go
into that
development
mentality and ask
yourself, "What
might I at any point
do
now with the assets
that I need to
upgrade myself at
present?" You
might have to do
more strength
preparation. You
might have to move
your preparation so
you're doing fewer
miles, yet better
quality miles.
There are dependable
steps you can take to
develop from where
you
are.

5. Compose another self-talk script.
We can be quite unforgiving with ourselves while we're encountering ourselves. At the point when all else fails, bombs have a go at saying, "That's right. This is hard. In any case, I got this: changes and challenges in our presentation. This is a great chance to rehearse some mental social treatment and catch yourself when those contemplations creep in and inquire, "Is this something I would agree to with another female?" The response is possible: "No, I wouldn't agree with that with anyone. That is not useful. It's not good. It's not humane. Furthermore,

it's positively not useful." So how might you address yourself in the future?

CHAPTER 9

MENOPAUSE AT WORK AND HOME

Survival methods

It's memorable that the menopause is typical and that help ought to be accessible to help you at work. Menopausal ladies are the quickest developing segment in the labor force, so it's significant now like never before to have the option to talk transparently about menopause at work. Menopause can influence a lady's functioning life. Once in a while

Menopausal side
effects or working
circumstances can
affect your
capacity to think or
complete your job
overall quite well.
Numerous ladies
have said that they
frequently find
dealing with their
Menopause side
effects in the
working environment
are extremely
testing.
Adapting to side
effects in the
working environment
can be
hard,particularly as
numerous ladies find
it challenging to
discuss
menopause at work.
Things you can do
You can demand
sensible changes be
made inside your
working
environment to assist
you with dealing

with your
menopausal side
effects,
For
example,adaptable
working,mentioning
an alternate uniform
on the
off chance that you
are encountering hot
flushes.
Moving to a cooler
piece of the
workplace or
requesting a
fanUtilizing
innovation where it
can help you, for
instance setting up
updates
on your telephone or
taking more notes to
assist with 'cerebrum
haze'.
It's valuable to
contemplate the
commonsense
changes that will
help
you.
Assuming you
approach a word

related wellbeing
administration, you
can address them
about help and
conceivable work
changes.
Assuming you have
strong work partners
and discuss your
encounters
with them, you might
observe that you're in
good company.
Beyond the working
environment, you
ought to consider
lifestyle
changes like
participating in more
activities or strolling
more as well as
eating a solid
adjusted diet. .

**How your manager
can uphold you**
Assuming you are
encountering
menopausal side
effects that are
influencing your
capacity to work,
you can address your
supervisor

and let them in on
the thing you're
going through.
Opening up to
somebody in an
expert climate might
feel off-kilter,
particularly on the
off chance that your
director is somebody
you feel
awkward conversing
with private matters.
In the event that you
feel
like this is the
situation, you could
take a stab at
addressing an
alternate
individual from your
supervisory crew or
HR (HR).
Prior to addressing
somebody you could
attempt.
Taking notes of your
menopausal side
effects and how or
when they
are influencing you.
Getting ready what
you intend to

examine with a
companion
Consider
arrangements that
you think could help
you. in the event that
you are a chief.
There are heaps of
assets accessible that
can assist you with
seeing
more about the
menopause and the
help ladies
encountering
menopausal side
effects in your work
environment may
need. There are
arrangements
accessible to assist
ladies with
proceeding to work
serenely during
menopause.

CHAPTER 10

LIFE   PAST
MENOPAUSE

Observing your excursion

1.Make the way of life change.
Numerous side effects can be just a result of changing things in your day-to-day existence. Eat a solid eating routine. Work-out routinely.
Quit smoking. Stop or break the point of your drinking. Everything
will help your general well-being while at the same time easing side effects and reducing your risk for future medical conditions. Side effects can be managed in a lot of ways. Above all, you really
 Want to visit your PCP to analyze menopause. Your side effects, age, and clinical history might be sufficient to

draw the conclusion.
If not,
Your PCP can run a
blood test to check
your chemical levels.
When
you have the
authority and
determination, you
can work with your
PCP
to foster an
arrangement to deal
with your side
effects.
Estrogen is normally
present in numerous
food sources; your
ovaries
aren't the main
source. So you can
enhance a solid,
plant-based diet
with these food
varieties to assist
with raising your
chemical levels; a
significant number of
them you
presumably eat as of
now:
Dried leafy foods:
organic products like

apricots, oranges,
strawberries,
and
peaches,Numerous
veggies, including
sweet potatoes,
carrots,
horse-feed
,fledglings, kale and
celery
Tofu and other soy-
based items.
Beans and lentils
Olives and olive oil
Flax and sesame
seeds
Spices like thyme,
sage, and turmeric
Notice the triggers of
your hot glimmers
and attempt to
oversee them.
Normal triggers
incorporate pressure,
heat, tobacco smoke,
liquor,
caffeine, tight attire,
and hot food sources.
On the off chance
that you experience
difficulty controlling
your

triggers, your PCP
can recommend
estrogen and
progesterone
medicines to up your
chemical levels.
Other doctors
prescribed drugs
like antidepressants,
anti seizure
medications, and
circulatory strain
meds can likewise
help.
These medicines can
likewise mitigate
different side effects,
including
emotional episodes,
sadness, and
nervousness.
2.Revive your vagina
At the point when
the demonstration of
sex is discomforting,
its
possibility is as well.
However, sex may
really save your
vagina.
Sexual movement
increases

bloodstream to the
area, assisting with
keeping it greased
up, protecting the
vaginal covering and
keeping it
from contracting.
Over-the-counter
vaginal ointments
and physician
recommended drugs
can likewise alleviate
the dryness and make
sex more agreeable
until
your vagina can
deliver enough all
alone.
Assuming you've
attempted everything
regardless of feeling
a steady
inconvenience, there
are further developed
other options. In a
speedy,
five-minute non-
hormonal treatment,
laser treatment
invigorates the
vaginal tissue to
deliver collagen,

further develop
usefulness and
reestablish harmony
to the mucous film.
Laser meetings are
under 5
minutes each and are
helpfully performed
solidly in the
workplace
during a standard
short term
arrangement.
At the point when
your ovaries tap out,
you shouldn't need
to. Low
estrogen levels
destroy your energy
and your personal
satisfaction.
Grasp your side
effects, get familiar
with your choices
and converse
with your medical
doctor.

CONCLUSIO
N

Your menopause, your way

All ladies go through menopause eventually in their lives. Individual

encounters with menopause vary massively, and how ladies decide to

deal with their menopause will depend upon various

variables,including age at menopause, the presence of any side effects,

and what these mean sfor their personal satisfaction. Risk factors for

cardiovascular illness, disease, and

osteoporosis will
likewise

illuminate their
choices. A few ladies
like to

take a more "normal"
way to deal with
menopause, while
certain ladies

will decide to utilize
chemical substitution
treatment (HRT).

For all ladies, dietary
and way of life
estimates have a
significant

impact, especially in
the menopausal
years, in lessening
side effects,

advancing general
prosperity, and
decreasing the
dangers of

unexpected issues.

Ladies ought to
subsequently
guarantee that they
have satisfactory

activity and a sound
eating routine as a
feature of
menopause.